HOW TO HAVE A HEALTHY PREGNANCY 101:

Essential Tips for Expecting Mothers

Empowering Expectant Moms with Evidence-Based Guidance for a Safe and Confident Pregnancy Journey

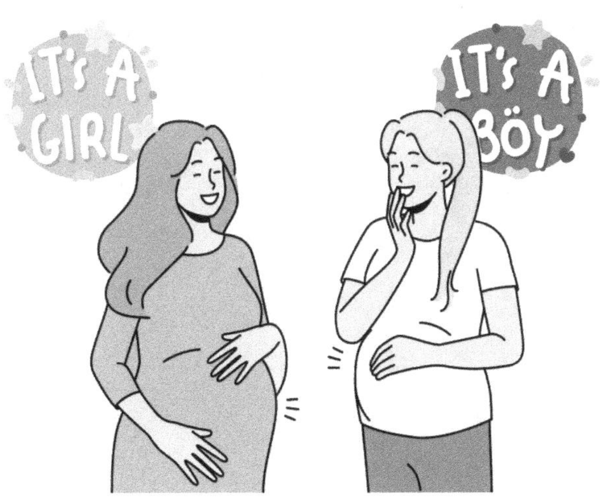

Peggy P. Rexford

TABLE OF CONTENTS

Introduction

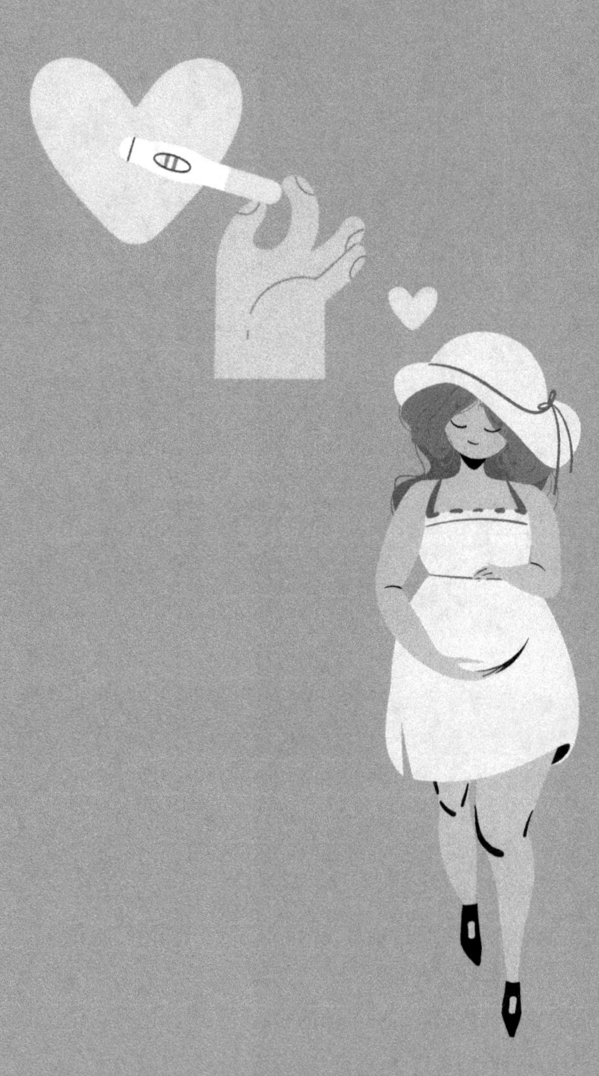

INTRODUCTION

Expecting a child is a wonderful and life-changing experience, but it also raises a slew of concerns, doubts, and problems.

In this book, we have compiled a variety of important insights, professional guidance, and practical recommendations to help you on your way to a healthy and enjoyable pregnancy. Each chapter is precisely designed to meet the specific needs and concerns of pregnant moms like you, from comprehending the physiological changes your body goes through to making educated decisions about nutrition, exercise, and self-care.

Whether you're a first-time parent or returning to the pregnant journey, this book will be your trusty companion every step of the way. With our help, you'll discover how to improve your health, nurture your growing baby, and embrace parenthood with grace and confidence.

Prepare to begin on an incredible journey to a beautiful and healthy pregnancy. Let us go on this journey together, because every woman deserves to feel powerful, knowledgeable, and supported on her path to parenthood.

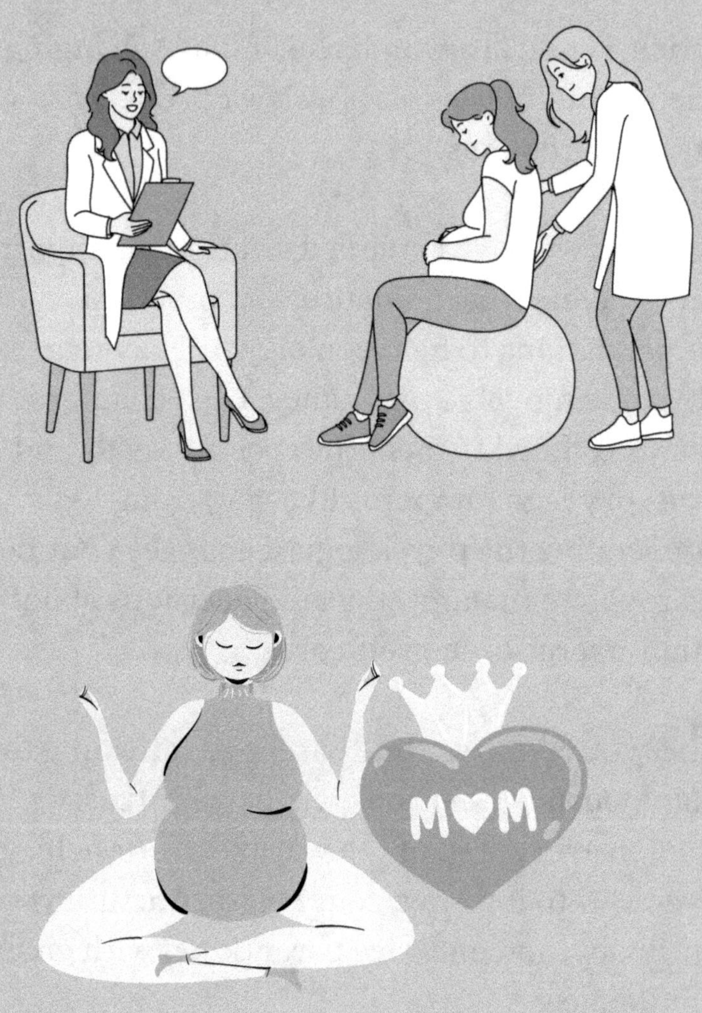

M♥M

CHAPTER ONE
Understanding the Basics of Pregnancy

The phases of pregnancy are usually separated into three trimesters, each lasting around three months. Here is a summary of each stage:

First trimester (weeks 1–12):

Conception happens when a sperm fertilizes an egg to generate a zygote.
The fertilized egg implants in the uterus, and the embryo starts to develop.
Major organs and body systems, including the heart, brain, and limbs, begin to develop.
Common symptoms include morning sickness, tiredness, breast soreness, and frequent urination.
By the conclusion of the first trimester, the embryo is formally classified as a fetus, and many pregnant moms have their first prenatal visits and tests.

Second trimester (weeks 13–26):

The fetus grows and develops quickly, with its organs growing and becoming more functional.
Most pregnant moms notice a decrease in early pregnancy symptoms, such as morning sickness, and may begin to feel more active.
Around the halfway of the second trimester, the mother begins to observe the baby's movements, known as quickening.
Many prenatal tests and screenings, including ultrasound scans, may be performed at this time to monitor the baby's growth and identify any possible problems.
Third trimester (weeks 27–40):

The fetus grows and develops rapidly, with a primary concentration on weight gain and preparation for delivery.
Expectant moms may suffer pain as their baby grows in size and puts pressure on their organs, resulting in symptoms including backaches, puffiness, and difficulties sleeping.
As the due date approaches, delivery preparations, such as attending prenatal courses and developing a birth plan, become more urgent.

Toward the conclusion of the third trimester, the baby may settle into a head-down position in preparation for delivery, though this might change.

Understanding the phases of pregnancy enables pregnant moms to monitor their baby's progress, predict changes in their bodies, and plan for the various milestones and challenges that lie ahead.

Important physiological changes during pregnancy

During pregnancy, a woman's body goes through several physiological changes that help the fetus grow and thrive. Some important physiological changes include:

Hormonal Changes:

Increased hormone levels, such as estrogen and progesterone, aid in pregnancy maintenance and fetal growth.

Hormonal shifts can cause symptoms including morning sickness, mood swings, and appetite changes.

- Cardiovascular Changes: To deliver nutrition and oxygen to the developing fetus, blood volume increases dramatically, by up to 50% over pre-pregnancy levels. The heart rate rises to match the increased blood volume, resulting in a quicker resting heart rate. Blood pressure may decline somewhat during early pregnancy before gradually returning to pre-pregnancy norms.
- Respiratory Changes: The expanding uterus exerts pressure on the diaphragm and lungs, causing shortness of breath and increased respiratory rate. Hormonal fluctuations can produce nasal congestion and increased mucus production, resulting in a sense of stuffiness.
- Renal Changes:Increased blood volume and hormonal changes cause increased blood flow to the kidneys, which leads to higher urine output. The kidneys work harder to filter waste from the mother's blood and eliminate it via urine.
- Gastrointestinal Changes: Hormonal changes and uterine growth pressure can cause gastrointestinal symptoms such nausea, vomiting, heartburn, and constipation. The digestive process may lag, resulting in delayed stomach emptying and stool motions.

Musculoskeletal Changes:

The body produces hormones such as relaxin, which relaxes the ligaments and joints in preparation for delivery, resulting in enhanced flexibility but also an increased chance of injury.
The enlarging uterus and weight growth might alter posture, resulting in back pain and discomfort.
Metabolic Changes:

The body's metabolism accelerates to meet the energy requirements of the developing baby and placenta. Insulin sensitivity may diminish, increasing the risk of gestational diabetes in certain women.
Understanding these physiological changes can assist pregnant moms in recognizing normal pregnancy symptoms, monitoring their health, and seeking medical assistance as needed. Regular prenatal care is crucial, as is communicating any concerns with healthcare experts to promote a healthy pregnancy for both mother and baby.

The importance of prenatal care and regular check-ups

Prenatal care and frequent check-ups throughout pregnancy are critical to ensure the health and well-being of both the mother and the developing baby. Here are some major reasons why prenatal care is important:

- Regular prenatal check-ups allow healthcare experts to monitor the mother's health throughout the pregnancy. This involves monitoring her weight increase, blood pressure, and overall health. Monitoring maternal health can aid in identifying and addressing possible problems or health concerns at an early stage.
- Monitoring Fetal Development: As part of prenatal care, the fetus's growth and development are monitored by frequent ultrasounds and screenings. These tests can help identify any anomalies or developmental concerns that may necessitate medical attention. Monitoring fetal growth also enables healthcare practitioners to change treatment plans as required to provide the best potential results for the infant.
- Preventing and Managing problems: Prenatal care aids in the identification and management of pregnancy-related problems or health concerns. For example, screening tests for gestational diabetes, preeclampsia, and other diseases can assist healthcare practitioners in intervening early to prevent difficulties and promote a safe pregnancy for both mother and baby.

Providing Education and Support: Prenatal care appointments allow pregnant women to receive education and support from healthcare professionals. This might include information on diet, fitness, birthing preparation, nursing, and infant care. Access to reliable information and assistance may help expecting moms make educated decisions, as well as feel more confident and prepared for childbirth and motherhood.

Establishing Relationships with Healthcare Providers: Prenatal care appointments help pregnant moms to build a connection with their healthcare professionals, such as obstetricians, midwives, or family doctors. Building trust and rapport with healthcare practitioners allows for open communication and ensures that pregnant women feel comfortable sharing any concerns or questions they may have during their pregnancy.

Overall, prenatal care and regular check-ups are critical in supporting a healthy pregnancy and achieving the best potential outcomes for both mother and baby. To get the most out of their prenatal treatment, pregnant women should attend all planned visits and talk honestly with their healthcare professionals.

Common myths and misconceptions regarding pregnancy

There are some prevalent pregnancy myths and misunderstandings that can cause undue anxiety or confusion for expecting mothers. Here are some of the most common myths.

Myth No. 1: "You should eat for two during pregnancy."

Fact: While it is necessary to consume more calories during pregnancy to assist fetal growth and development, the term "eating for two" is incorrect. Most women only need to increase their calorie intake by a little amount, often 300-500 calories per day, depending on their pre-pregnancy weight and activity level.

Myth says, "You shouldn't dye your hair or paint your nails during pregnancy."

While it is typically suggested to avoid some chemical exposures during pregnancy, such as those present in hair dyes and nail polishes, there is minimal evidence that even occasional use of these items provides substantial dangers to the developing fetus. If you have any worries, it is always best to choose safer, non-toxic alternatives or talk with a healthcare expert.

Myth #1: "You should avoid all seafood during pregnancy."

Fact: While high-mercury fish including shark, swordfish, king mackerel, and tilefish should be avoided during pregnancy, many other forms of seafood are safe and healthful. Fish and shellfish have high levels of omega-3 fatty acids, which are necessary for prenatal brain and eye development. It is suggested to eat low-mercury foods like salmon, shrimp, and trout, and to minimize eating of high-mercury seafood.

Myth No. 1: "You shouldn't travel or fly during pregnancy."

Fact: It is generally safe for pregnant women to travel and fly throughout pregnancy, particularly during the second trimester, when the risk of difficulties is reduced. However, it is critical to exercise caution, such as staying hydrated, using compression stockings to lower the chance of blood clots, and taking regular pauses to walk about and stretch during lengthy flights or vehicle journeys.

Myth No. 1: "You can predict the baby's gender based on certain pregnancy symptoms or old wives' tales."

CHAPTER TWO
Nutrition & Diet during Pregnancy.

A healthy pregnancy necessitates a well-balanced diet rich in critical nutrients to support both the mother's health and the baby' growth and development. Here are some essential nutrients that are especially vital during pregnancy:

Folic Acid (Folate): Folic acid is essential for avoiding neural tube disorders like spina bifida in the growing fetus. It is suggested that all women of childbearing age ingest 400-800 micrograms (mcg) of folic acid per day, beginning before conception and continuing throughout the first trimester of pregnancy.

Iron: Iron is required for red blood cell production and to avoid anemia, which is frequent during pregnancy owing to increased blood volume. Pregnant women require around 27 milligrams (mg) of iron per day, which may be supplied from foods including lean meats, chicken, fish, beans, fortified cereals, and dark leafy greens.

Calcium: Both the mother and the developing baby require calcium to create strong bones and teeth. Pregnant women should aim for 1,000-1,300 milligrams (mg) of calcium per day, which can be obtained from dairy products, fortified plant-based milks, tofu, almonds, and leafy greens.

Omega-3 Fatty Acids: Omega-3 fatty acids, particularly DHA (docosahexaenoic acid), are essential for the development of the embryonic brain and eyes. Pregnant women should strive to get at least 200-300 milligrams (mg) of DHA per day, which may be found in fatty fish like salmon, trout, and sardines, as well as walnuts, flaxseeds, and fortified meals.

Protein is necessary for the growth and development of the fetus and placenta, as well as the mother's health. Pregnant women should aim to take around 71 grams of protein per day, which can come from lean meats, poultry, fish, eggs, dairy products, legumes, and tofu.

Vitamin D: Vitamin D is essential for calcium absorption and bone health in both the mother and the growing child. Pregnant women should eat 600-800 International Units (IU) of vitamin D per day, which can be acquired via fortified meals, fatty fish, eggs, and sunshine.

Vitamin C is essential for maintaining the immune system and boosting iron absorption from plant-based sources. Pregnant women should have at least 85 milligrams (mg) of vitamin C per day, which may be found in citrus fruits, strawberries, kiwi, bell peppers, and broccoli.

In addition to these vital nutrients, pregnant women should keep hydrated by drinking enough of water and eat a range of nutrient-dense meals from all food groups to satisfy their increased nutritional requirements during pregnancy. For specialized dietary advice and assistance throughout pregnancy, speak with a healthcare professional or a certified dietitian.

Foods to avoid when pregnant.

During pregnancy, it is essential to avoid some meals that may be harmful to both the mother and the growing fetus. Here are some foods you should avoid or restrict during pregnancy.

Consuming raw or undercooked meat, poultry, and seafood raises the risk of foodborne infections such salmonella, listeria, and toxoplasmosis. Make certain that all meat, poultry, and fish are fully cooked to eliminate any hazardous germs or parasites.

Raw or undercooked eggs may contain salmonella bacteria, which can lead to food poisoning. Avoid eating items with raw or undercooked eggs, such as homemade Caesar salad dressing, hollandaise sauce, and uncooked cookie dough.

Unpasteurized dairy products, such as raw milk and some soft cheeses, may contain hazardous germs like listeria, which can result in miscarriage, stillbirth, or other major health concerns. To lessen the risk of foodborne disease, use pasteurized dairy products.

Unwashed Fruits and veggies: Before eating fruits and veggies, fully wash them to eliminate dirt, germs, and pesticide residues. Properly washing fruits and vegetables can help lower the risk of foodborne disease.

Rich-Mercury Fish: Certain species of fish, such as shark, swordfish, king mackerel, and tilefish, are rich in mercury, which can impair the developing neural system of the fetus. Limit your consumption of high-mercury seafood and instead choose for low-mercury choices like salmon, trout, shrimp, and canned light tuna.

Raw sprouts, including alfalfa, clover, and radish sprouts, can be infected with hazardous pathogens like salmonella and E. coli. To lessen the risk of foodborne disease, avoid eating raw sprouts and instead fully boil them before eating.

Excessive Caffeine: High caffeine intake during pregnancy has been linked to an increased risk of miscarriage and low birth weight. Limit your caffeine intake to no more than 200 milligrams per day, which is about comparable to one 12-ounce cup of coffee.

Alcohol intake during pregnancy has been linked to fetal alcohol spectrum disorders (FASDs), which can result in lifelong physical, behavioral, and intellectual problems in the newborn. Avoid consuming alcohol completely throughout pregnancy to safeguard the baby's health and well-being.

Avoiding these items and adopting smart dietary choices during pregnancy will help you and your baby have a safe and successful pregnancy. For specialized dietary advice and assistance throughout pregnancy, speak with a healthcare professional or a certified dietitian.

Meal planning and balanced diet

Here's a recommended meal plan and balanced diet throughout pregnancy to help you and your baby get the nutrients they need for a healthy pregnancy:

Breakfast:

Whole grain cereal, milk, and sliced strawberries
Hard-boiled egg.
Whole wheat toast with avocado spread.
For more calcium and vitamin D, try orange juice or fortified plant-based milk.

Snack:

Greek yogurt and mixed fruit
A handful of almonds or walnuts for extra protein and healthy fats.
Carrot sticks with hummus are a crisp and healthful snack.

Lunch:

Grilled chicken or tofu salad topped with mixed greens, cherry tomatoes, cucumber, and feta cheese.
Quinoa or brown rice pilaf with roasted veggies (such as bell peppers, zucchini, and onions).
Whole grain wrap filled with lean turkey, spinach, avocado, and mustard.

Snack:

Apple slices and peanut butter
Cottage cheese with pineapple chunks
Whole grain crackers with sliced cheese

Dinner:

Baked salmon, steamed broccoli, and quinoa
Stir-fried tofu with mixed veggies (e.g., bell peppers, snap peas, and carrots), served over brown rice
Lentil soup served with whole grain bread and a side salad.

Snack/Dessert:

Banana smoothie with Greek yogurt, spinach, and almond milk.
Whole grain toast with almond butter and sliced banana.
Dark chocolate-dipped strawberries are a tasty delicacy (in moderation).

Hydration:

Drink lots of water all day to keep hydrated. Aim for at least 8 to 10 glasses of water every day.
Limit your intake of caffeinated beverages and replace them with decaffeinated tea or coffee as needed.
Consider using herbal drinks like ginger or peppermint for nausea relief, but see your doctor first. Remember to include diversity, balance, and moderation in your meals. To ensure you satisfy your nutritional needs, consume a variety of protein, carbs, healthy fats, fruits, and vegetables in each meal. Listen to your body's hunger and fullness cues, and get tailored meal planning assistance from your healthcare practitioner or a qualified dietitian while pregnant.

Addressing cravings and regulating weight gain.

Addressing cravings and maintaining weight gain during pregnancy necessitates a balanced strategy that considers both the mother's and the growing baby's nutritional needs. Here are some strategies to help with cravings and managing weight gain during pregnancy:

Understanding Cravings: Pregnancy cravings are frequent and can be triggered by hormonal shifts, dietary deficits, or just a need for comfort foods. It's critical to acknowledge that occasional cravings are OK, but strive to make healthier choices whenever feasible.

Choose Nutrient-Dense meals: Rather than giving in to cravings for unhealthy or processed meals, attempt to fulfill them with nutrient-dense options. For example, if you're desiring something sweet, try fresh fruit or a tiny amount of dark chocolate.

Allow yourself to indulge in desires on occasion, but practice moderation to avoid excessive weight gain and maintain a healthy diet. Consider portion management and mindful eating practices to help you manage urges without overeating.

Stay Hydrated: Thirst is sometimes confused with hunger or desires. Drink lots of water throughout the day to keep hydrated and reduce cravings. Choose water or other hydrating liquids over sugary drinks or sodas.

Incorporate Balanced Meals: Make an effort to include meals and snacks that contain a variety of protein, carbs, healthy fats, fruits, and vegetables. Eating balanced meals can assist to regulate blood sugar levels and minimize the severity of cravings.

Stay Active: Engaging in regular physical exercise throughout pregnancy can help manage weight gain, enhance mood, and decrease cravings. Walking, swimming, or pregnant yoga are all low-impact workouts that your healthcare practitioner may approve of.

Listen to your body. Pay attention to your body's hunger and fullness cues; eat when you're hungry, and stop when you're full. Avoid missing meals or depriving yourself of food, since this might result in extreme desires and overeating later.

Seek Help: If you're having trouble managing cravings or weight gain throughout your pregnancy, speak with your doctor or a certified dietitian. They can offer tailored advice and assistance to help you make healthy choices and eat a balanced diet.

Remember that weight growth is a natural and important aspect of pregnancy, but it's critical to aim for moderate and consistent weight gain within the suggested range. Focus on fueling your body with good meals, being active, and listening to your body's requirements to ensure a successful pregnancy for both you and your child.

Dietary recommendations during distinct stages of pregnancy

There are unique dietary concerns for each stage of pregnancy that can assist support the changing requirements of both the mother and the developing baby. Here are some specific dietary recommendations for each stage of pregnancy:

First trimester (weeks 1–12):

To manage nausea and morning sickness, eat small, frequent meals throughout the day and avoid strong-smelling or fatty foods.
To assist neural tube development, ensure an appropriate intake of folic acid-rich meals or supplements.
Stay hydrated, since dehydration can worsen nausea and exhaustion.
Include high-fiber meals to aid with constipation, which is a typical complaint in early pregnancy.
Second trimester (weeks 13–26):

Continue to prioritize nutrient-dense meals to promote fetal growth and development.
Increase your consumption of iron-rich meals to help increase your blood volume and avoid anemia.
Incorporate calcium-rich meals to help the baby's bone and tooth growth.
Consider include omega-3 fatty acids in your baby's diet to help with brain and eye development.

Third trimester (weeks 27–40):
Ensure a enough protein intake to promote the baby's growth and development, particularly during the fast growth phase in the third trimester.
Monitor fluid consumption to avoid dehydration and maintain amniotic fluid levels.
Consume vitamin K-rich meals to help with blood clotting before delivery.
Incorporate antioxidant-rich meals, such as fruits and vegetables, to boost immune function and decrease inflammation.
During Pregnancy:

Aim for a well-balanced diet rich in nutrients from all food categories.
To satisfy increased nutritional demands, eat lean protein, entire grains, fruits, vegetables, and healthy fats.
Avoid or minimize processed meals, sugary snacks, and excessive caffeine consumption.
Discuss any dietary limitations or concerns with your doctor or a certified dietitian to ensure you're getting enough nutrients.
Throughout your pregnancy, pay attention to your body's hunger and fullness cues and change your diet as needed. Furthermore, speaking with a healthcare professional or a certified dietitian may give tailored advice and support to help you make smart food choices and promote a successful pregnancy for both you and your baby.

Third trimester (weeks 27–40):

Ensure a enough protein intake to promote the baby's growth and development, particularly during the fast growth phase in the third trimester.

Monitor fluid consumption to avoid dehydration and maintain amniotic fluid levels.

Consume vitamin K-rich meals to help with blood clotting before delivery.

Incorporate antioxidant-rich meals, such as fruits and vegetables, to boost immune function and decrease inflammation.

During Pregnancy:

Aim for a well-balanced diet rich in nutrients from all food categories.

To satisfy increased nutritional demands, eat lean protein, entire grains, fruits, vegetables, and healthy fats.

Avoid or minimize processed meals, sugary snacks, and excessive caffeine consumption.

Discuss any dietary limitations or concerns with your doctor or a certified dietitian to ensure you're getting enough nutrients.

Throughout your pregnancy, pay attention to your body's hunger and fullness cues and change your diet as needed. Furthermore, speaking with a healthcare professional or a certified dietitian may give tailored advice and support to help you make smart food choices and promote a successful pregnancy for both you and your baby.

CHAPTER THREE
Exercise and Physical Activity for Expectant Mothers

Exercise during pregnancy has several benefits to both the mother and the growing baby. Some of the main advantages of exercising during pregnancy include:

Improved Physical Health: Regular exercise throughout pregnancy can assist to enhance cardiovascular health, maintain muscular tone and strength, and boost overall stamina and endurance. It also helps to avoid excessive weight gain and lowers the chance of developing gestational diabetes and high blood pressure.

Reduced Discomfort: Exercise can assist with typical pregnant symptoms including back pain, edema, constipation, and bloating. Strengthening and stretching exercises can help improve posture and reduce muscular tension, resulting in more comfort and mobility.

Better Mood and Mental Health: Exercise produces endorphins, which are natural mood enhancers that assist to alleviate stress, anxiety, and depression during pregnancy. Regular physical activity can enhance sleep quality, self-esteem, and overall well-being.

Enhanced Sleep: Regular exercise can help regulate sleep patterns and increase sleep quality when pregnant. However, strenuous activity should be avoided close to bedtime to minimize sleep interruptions.

Preparation for Labor and Delivery: Exercise develops the muscles required for labor and delivery, especially the pelvic floor. It can also boost endurance and stamina, which are useful for the physical demands of labor.

Women who exercise throughout pregnancy often have a speedier postpartum recovery, including a quicker return to pre-pregnancy weight, greater muscle tone, and a lower risk of postpartum depression.

Positive Impact on Fetal Development: Studies show that maternal activity during pregnancy may promote fetal development by improving fetal heart rate variability, lowering birth weight, and lowering the risk of obesity and chronic illnesses later in life.

Bonding and Connection: Exercise can help expecting moms connect with their bodies and their developing baby. Prenatal yoga and swimming are two activities that might help mothers and babies relax and bond.

Safe and recommended workouts for pregnant women

Pregnant women can safely participate in a range of workouts during their pregnancy, as long as they have approval from their healthcare practitioner and listen to their bodies. Below are some safe and suggested workouts for pregnant women:

Walking is a low-impact workout that is suitable for all stages of pregnancy. It promotes cardiovascular health, muscular tone, and general stamina. Aim for 30 minutes of brisk walking most days of the week.

Swimming and water aerobics are ideal alternatives for pregnant women because they give a full-body exercise while minimizing joint stress. The buoyancy of water relieves strain on the back and joints and might give the sensation of weightlessness.

Prenatal yoga emphasizes moderate stretching, relaxation, and breathing techniques, making it appropriate for pregnant women. It improves flexibility, strength, and balance while also promoting relaxation and stress reduction.

Stationary cycling or indoor cycling sessions are suitable for pregnant women since they give a low-impact cardiovascular workout. Adjust the resistance and tempo to your comfort level, and avoid exercises that involve abrupt or jarring movements.

Low-impact aerobics programs tailored to pregnant women can provide a safe and efficient workout. To reduce the chance of injury, avoid high-impact motions, leaping, and quick direction changes.

Strength Training: Resistance bands, small weights, or bodyweight workouts can help you maintain muscular tone and strength while pregnant. Concentrate on exercises that work key muscular groups, such as squats, lunges, bicep curls, and shoulder presses.

Pelvic floor exercises, also known as Kegel exercises, aim to strengthen the pelvic floor muscles, which helps support the uterus, bladder, and intestines during pregnancy while also improving bladder control. Kegel exercises should be practiced on a regular basis during pregnancy.

Always warm up before working out, remain hydrated, and listen to your body. Avoid laying flat on your back after the first trimester, since this might reduce blood supply to the uterus. If you feel any discomfort, pain, dizziness, or strange symptoms while exercising, stop immediately and visit your doctor.

Precautions and adaptations during the various trimesters

Precautions and adjustments for exercising during pregnancy vary per trimester. Below are some broad rules for each trimester:

- First trimester (weeks 1–12):
- Precautions: Avoid overheating as it might damage the growing fetus. Avoid exercising in hot or humid weather, and remain hydrated.
- Listen to your body and avoid activities that make you uncomfortable or tired.
- Exercises that require you to lie flat on your back for a lengthy amount of time should be avoided since they might reduce blood supply to the uterus.

Modifications: Reduce intensity if feeling nausea, tiredness, or dizziness.

Choose low-impact activities like walking, swimming, or prenatal yoga.
Gentle stretching and relaxation exercises might help ease early pregnancy discomfort.

Second trimester (weeks 13–26):

To reduce the chance of injury, avoid activities involving rapid changes in direction, leaping, or high-impact motions.
Exercises requiring balance should be performed with caution since your center of gravity may alter as your belly expands.
Stay hydrated and prevent overheating when exercising.

Modifications:
Modify abdominal workouts to prevent resting flat on your back. Instead, perform workouts while reclining or resting on your side.
Wearing a belly support band or pregnancy support belt can provide additional comfort and support while exercising.
Choose workouts that help to retain strength and flexibility, such as prenatal Pilates or swimming.

Third trimester (weeks 27–40):

Precautions: Avoid abdominal-pressure workouts like crunches and twisting.
Exercises on your hands and knees should be performed with caution, since this posture may become unpleasant as your tummy swells.
Stay hydrated and take breaks when necessary to relax and recuperate during activity.
Modifications: Practice relaxation activities, such prenatal yoga or mild stretching, to prepare the body for labor and delivery.
To decrease joint and ligament tension, engage in low-impact exercises such as walking, swimming, or stationary cycling.
Listen to your body and adapt your workout intensity and duration as needed to compensate for weariness and discomfort.
Regardless of trimester, you should contact with your doctor before beginning or maintaining an exercise regimen during pregnant. They can make unique suggestions based on your specific health state and pregnancy demands. Remember to listen to your body, remain hydrated, and adjust workouts as required to maintain a safe and enjoyable workout throughout your pregnancy.

Using relaxation methods and stress management

Incorporating relaxation methods and stress management measures into your daily routine will help you feel better overall throughout pregnancy. Here are several methods pregnant women may implement relaxation techniques and stress management:

Deep Breathing: Deep breathing techniques can help you relax and reduce tension. Take slow, deep breathes in through your nose and exhale through your mouth. Concentrate on filling your lungs with air and releasing tension with each inhalation.

Mindfulness Meditation: Practice mindfulness meditation to increase present-moment awareness and lower stress. Find a peaceful place, sit comfortably, and concentrate on your breathing or a specific sensation in your body. Allow ideas to pass without judgment, restoring your attention to the present moment.

Progressive Muscle Relaxation: To practice progressive muscle relaxation, methodically tens and releases different muscle groups throughout your body. Begin with your toes and work your way up to your head, tensing each muscle group for a few seconds before letting go and relaxing entirely.

Yoga: Take a prenatal yoga class or practice at home with prenatal yoga DVDs. Yoga may help you improve your flexibility, strength, and balance while also promoting relaxation and stress reduction via moderate stretching and breathing techniques.

Guided Imagery: Using guided imagery or visualization techniques, build a mental image of a tranquil and relaxing environment. Close your eyes, envision yourself in a peaceful setting, and concentrate on all of the sensory aspects, including sights, sounds, scents, and textures.

Massage treatment: Prenatal massage treatment can help you ease muscular tension, reduce stress, and relax. Look for a professional massage therapist who specializes in prenatal massage and express any specific concerns or pain.

Self-Care Activities: Do things that make you happy and relax, such as reading, listening to music, having a warm bath, or spending time in nature. Make self-care a priority by setting aside time for activities that feed your body, mind, and spirit.

Seek help from family, friends, or pregnancy support organizations. Sharing your ideas and feelings with people who understand what you're going through may bring you comfort, validation, and support at difficult times.

Tips for being active and maintaining fitness levels when pregnant

Here are some ways to assist pregnant women keep active and include exercise into their daily routine:

Consult Your Healthcare Provider: Before beginning or maintaining an exercise regimen during pregnancy, check with your doctor to confirm that it is safe for you and your baby. Your healthcare professional can make unique suggestions based on your specific health state and pregnancy requirements.

Choose Safe and Low-Impact Activities: Pregnancy-friendly activities include strolling, swimming, stationary cycling, prenatal yoga, and water aerobics. These exercises promote cardiovascular health, maintain muscular tone, and alleviate stress without putting undue strain on joints and ligaments.

Listen to Your Body: Pay attention to your body's cues and adjust or discontinue any activity that produces discomfort, pain, or weariness. Avoid pushing yourself too hard and instead emphasize your comfort and safety when exercising.

Stay Hydrated: Drink lots of water before, during, and after exercise to avoid overheating. Aim to drink water throughout the day, especially if you're doing vigorous exercise.

Warm-up and Cool Down: Always begin your workout session with a modest warm-up to prepare your body for action and lower your chance of injury. After exercise, cool down with stretching activities to help relax and extend your muscles.

Modify workouts as Needed: As your pregnancy continues, you may need to adjust your workouts to fit your growing body. Avoid workouts that require you to lie flat on your back after the first trimester, since this might reduce blood supply to the uterus. Listen to your body and make necessary modifications to guarantee a comfortable and safe workout.

Wear Comfortable and Supportive Clothing and Footwear: Choose clothing that allows for ease of movement and provides adequate support for your developing tummy. Invest in supportive footwear with strong arch support and cushioning to lessen the chance of foot and ankle discomfort when exercising.

Set Realistic objectives: Determine your current fitness level and pregnancy status to set realistic and achievable fitness objectives. Concentrate on maintaining your present fitness level rather than trying for huge increases, and enjoy your success along the way.

Be Consistent: Try to include regular physical activity into your daily routine, with at least 150 minutes of moderate-intensity exercise each week, as suggested by the American College of Obstetricians and Gynecologists (ACOG). Break your training sessions into shorter bursts if necessary, and prioritize consistency over intensity.

Seek Support and Accountability: To keep motivated and accountable to your fitness objectives, team up with a workout companion, enroll in a prenatal exercise class, or join online groups for pregnant women. Surround yourself with good influencers who will encourage and support your attempts to be active while pregnant.

Following these recommendations and guidelines can allow pregnant women to stay active, maintain fitness levels, and get the numerous advantages of exercise during their pregnancy. Remember to listen to your body, emphasize safety and comfort, and speak with your doctor if you have any questions or concerns about exercising while pregnant.

CHAPTER FOUR

Emotional Well-being and Self-Care during Pregnancy.

Understanding emotional shifts and mood swings during pregnancy is crucial for pregnant moms as they navigate this unique and often difficult time. Here are some tips for identifying and managing emotional shifts and mood swings when pregnant:

Hormonal swings: Hormonal alterations contribute significantly to emotional swings throughout pregnancy. Hormonal fluctuations, such as estrogen and progesterone, can influence neurotransmitters in the brain, resulting in mood swings, impatience, and emotional sensitivities.

Physical Discomfort: Nausea, exhaustion, back pain, and hunger changes can all contribute to emotional disturbances and mood swings. Physical pain can have an affect on one's mood and mental well-being.

Stress and Anxiety: Pregnancy can cause new tensions and worries due to changes in lifestyle, money, relationships, and concerns about birthing and parenthood. Managing stress and anxiety levels is critical to mental well-being throughout pregnancy.

Body Image and Self-Esteem: During pregnancy, changes in body shape, weight gain, and physical symptoms like swollen feet or stretch marks can all have an affect on body image and self-esteem. It is natural to have swings in body image and self-confidence as the body adjusts to accommodate the developing baby.

Pregnancy can impact relationships with partners, family members, and friends, causing changes in communication, intimacy, and support dynamics. Expectant moms may experience emotional highs and lows while navigating these relationship adjustments.

Coping skills: Learning good coping skills will help you handle emotional shifts and mood swings when pregnant. Mindfulness meditation, deep breathing exercises, writing, hobbies, and seeking assistance from loved ones can all help you cope with emotional ups and downs.

Seeking Support: When pregnant women experience emotional shifts and mood swings, they should seek help from their healthcare professionals, partners, family members, and friends. Talking freely about your thoughts and worries with trusted people may bring affirmation, comfort, and perspective.

Professional Help: If emotional changes and mood swings become overwhelming or interfere with everyday functioning, it may be helpful to seek professional assistance from a therapist, counselor, or mental health specialist. Therapy or therapy might help you manage your emotions throughout pregnancy.

Expectant women may manage the emotional journey of pregnancy with better ease and resilience by recognizing the elements that lead to emotional shifts and mood swings, as well as employing coping mechanisms and support networks. Remember that it is natural to feel a variety of emotions throughout pregnancy, and seeking help is a show of strength, not weakness.

Coping with stress and anxiety throughout pregnancy.

Coping with stress and anxiety during pregnancy is critical for the health of both the expecting woman and the baby. Pregnant women can utilize the following ways to manage stress and anxiety:

Incorporating relaxation techniques into your regular routine can help reduce stress and anxiety. Deep breathing techniques, gradual muscular relaxation, guided imagery, and mindfulness meditation all help to relax and calm the mind.

Stay Active: Regular physical activity can help decrease stress and enhance mood. Low-impact workouts like walking, swimming, prenatal yoga, and mild stretching can improve both physical and mental health.

Maintain a Healthy Lifestyle: Prioritize self-care by eating healthy meals, staying hydrated, getting enough sleep, and avoiding alcohol and tobacco. A healthy lifestyle can improve general well-being and reduce stress during pregnancy.

Create a Support System: Surround yourself with sympathetic and understanding people who can offer encouragement, empathy, and practical aid. During stressful or anxious situations, seek assistance from your partner, family members, friends, and healthcare providers.

Communicate Your Emotions: Share your ideas, feelings, and worries with your spouse, loved ones, or a reputable healthcare professional. Talking freely about your emotions might make you feel less isolated while also providing affirmation and support.

Practice mindfulness by staying present in the moment and focusing on what you can control. Mindfulness is paying nonjudgmental attention to your thoughts, feelings, and experiences. Mindfulness exercises can assist to alleviate anxiety and foster a sense of peace and acceptance.

Limit Stressor Exposure: Identify stressors in your life and take efforts to reduce your exposure to them as much as feasible. Set boundaries, delegate chores, and prioritize activities that provide joy and relaxation.

Seek Professional Help: If stress and anxiety become excessive or interfere with everyday functioning, do not be afraid to seek professional assistance from a therapist, counselor, or mental health specialist. Therapy or counseling can offer additional assistance and coping methods for stress and anxiety throughout pregnancy.

Remember that it is natural to feel stressed and anxious throughout pregnancy, but getting assistance and applying coping methods can help ease symptoms and improve mental health. Be proactive in managing stress, prioritize self-care, and seek help when necessary.

Importance of sufficient sleep and relaxation

Adequate sleep and relaxation are essential for good health and well-being, particularly during pregnancy. Here are some of the primary benefits of good sleep and relaxation:

Physical Health: Adequate sleep and relaxation help the body repair and rebuild cells, tissues, and muscles. Adequate rest strengthens the immune system, lowers blood pressure, and reduces the risk of chronic illnesses including heart disease and diabetes.

Mental Health: Sleep and relaxation are essential for preserving mental and emotional health. Adequate rest improves cognitive function, focus, and memory while also regulating mood and reducing stress. Lack of sleep and relaxation can exacerbate mood problems including sadness and anxiety.

Stress Reduction: Deep breathing, meditation, and mindfulness exercises can all assist to decrease stress and produce a sense of peace and relaxation. Adequate rest enables the body and mind to recuperate from everyday stresses and better deal with problems.

Improved Focus and Productivity: Adequate rest and relaxation are required for peak cognitive performance, focus, and productivity. Getting adequate sleep improves attention, problem-solving skills, and decision-making abilities, resulting in higher productivity and efficiency in everyday chores.

Hormonal Balance: Sleep and relaxation help to regulate the synthesis of hormones including cortisol, melatonin, and serotonin. Adequate rest promotes a healthy hormonal balance, which is essential for mood regulation, hunger management, and reproductive health.

Healthy Pregnancy: Adequate sleep and relaxation during pregnancy are especially crucial for the mother's and baby's health and well-being. Quality sleep promotes baby growth, immunological function, and mother health, while relaxing methods can alleviate typical pregnant symptoms including nausea, back pain, and insomnia.

Appetite and Weight Management: Sleep and relaxation help to regulate appetite hormones like leptin and ghrelin, which influence hunger and satiety. Adequate rest helps to reduce overeating and cravings for harmful foods, which can improve weight management and general health.

Improved Immune Function: Proper sleep and relaxation boost the immune system, allowing the body to fight off infections and diseases. Adequate rest stimulates the synthesis of immune cells and antibodies, lowering the risk of sickness and facilitating speedier recovery.

Overall, getting enough sleep and relaxation is critical for sustaining physical, mental, and emotional health and encouraging a healthy and balanced lifestyle, especially during pregnancy. Incorporating relaxation methods into your everyday routine, as well as creating a pleasant sleep environment, will help you feel better and support your pregnancy.

Creating a support network and getting expert assistance.

Self-care during pregnancy includes developing a support network and recognizing when to seek expert help. Pregnant women can take the following actions to develop a support network and get expert aid when necessary:

Identify Supportive People: Contact family members, friends, partners, coworkers, and other pregnant women who may provide emotional support, encouragement, and understanding during pregnancy. Surround yourself with supportive people who can offer emotional, practical, and social support.

Join Support Groups: Consider joining pregnant women's support groups or online communities to connect with others going through similar circumstances. These organizations may offer a sense of community, affirmation, and understanding, as well as helpful information and tools.

Attend Prenatal courses: Attend prenatal courses or seminars given by healthcare practitioners, community centers, or birthing facilities. Prenatal courses offer instruction, assistance, and support on issues like as childbirth, breastfeeding, baby care, and postpartum recovery, as well as the chance to meet other pregnant parents.

Communicate Openly: Tell your spouse, family members, and healthcare providers about your pregnancy-related thoughts, feelings, and worries. Effective communication promotes understanding, empathy, and support while also strengthening connections during this transitional period.

Seek Professional treatment: If you are suffering symptoms of depression, anxiety, or other mental health issues that are interfering with your daily functioning or quality of life, don't be afraid to seek professional treatment from a therapist, counselor, or mental health specialist. Therapy or counseling can offer extra support, coping methods, and treatment alternatives to help you deal with emotional difficulties throughout pregnancy.

Consult with Healthcare professionals: Keep open and honest communication with your healthcare professionals, such as your obstetrician, midwife, or doula, about any physical or emotional problems you may have during pregnancy. Your healthcare practitioners can give information, support, and recommendations to relevant resources and services as required.

Take proactive efforts to educate yourself about pregnancy, labor, postpartum recovery, and infant care by reading books, attending classes, and collecting information from reliable sources. Knowledge allows you to make more educated decisions and advocate for your own health and well-being.

Prioritize Self-Care: Make self-care a top priority by participating in activities that promote relaxation, stress reduction, and general well-being. Practice relaxing techniques such as deep breathing, meditation, yoga, or massage treatment, and set aside time for things that offer you joy and refreshment.

Pregnant women can better handle the emotional ups and downs of pregnancy by developing a strong support network, talking freely with loved ones and healthcare professionals, getting professional help when necessary, and emphasizing self-care. Remember that asking for help is OK, and that aid is there when you need it.

Bonding with your baby and getting ready for the adventure ahead.

Bonding with your baby throughout pregnancy is a lovely and crucial part of becoming a mother. Here are some ways pregnant women may bond with their baby and be ready for the road ahead:

Talk to Your kid: Begin chatting to your kid on a regular basis, even before birth. Share your thoughts, feelings, hopes, and dreams with your infant out loud. You may also entertain your infant by reading books, singing songs, or playing music.

Prenatal Yoga and Meditation: Practice prenatal yoga and meditation to bond with your baby and cultivate a sense of peace and serenity. These routines can help you connect with your body and your baby's movements, building a stronger link.

Create a Pregnancy notebook: Begin a pregnancy notebook to record your thoughts, experiences, and milestones during your pregnancy. Write messages to your kid, scribble down recollections, or record moments of happiness and anticipation.

Attend Prenatal Classes: Enroll in prenatal classes or seminars that give instruction and support to expecting moms. Classes on labor preparation, nursing, baby care, and postpartum recovery will help you feel more prepared and powerful as you embark on this journey.

Visualize Your Baby: Spend time each day imagining how your baby could look, sound, and feel. Imagine yourself holding your kid, caressing them, and caring for them once they're born.

Bond Through Touch: Use gentle touch and massage techniques on your tummy to bond with your baby. You may also invite your spouse to participate by putting their hand on your tummy and feeling for the baby's movements.

Create a Baby Registry: Begin planning for your baby's arrival by establishing a baby registry with the key goods you'll require. Shopping for baby clothes, nursery décor, and baby items may make you feel closer to your kid and more thrilled about their birth.

Attend sessions Together: Include your spouse in prenatal and ultrasound sessions whenever feasible. Seeing and hearing your baby's heartbeat and developmental milestones can help to enhance your family relationship.

Prepare the Nursery: Create a unique area in your house for your baby, whether it's a separate nursery or a comfortable nook of your bedroom. Decorating the nursery, arranging furniture, and organizing newborn supplies can make you feel more prepared and closer to your child.

Prioritize self-care activities that feed your body, mind, and spirit throughout pregnancy. Take some time to rest, relax, and recharge, remembering that caring for yourself is an important part of caring for your kid.

By taking deliberate measures to bond with your baby throughout pregnancy and prepare for the journey ahead, you may foster a deep connection and sense of anticipation for your child's birth. Enjoy every moment of this unique time and believe in the love and relationship that will develop between you and your kid long after they are born.